The Vibrant Mediterranean Side Dishes Recipe Book

A Complete Collection of Side Dishes to Boost Your Mediterranean Meals

Carl Ewing

Table of Contents

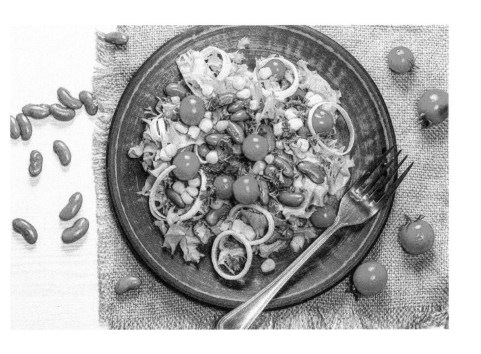

Pesto and Lemon Asparagus

Prep time: 10 minutes I **Cooking time:** 20 minutes I

Servings: 4

Ingredients:

- 1 pound asparagus, trimmed
- 2 tablespoons basil pesto
- 1 tablespoon lemon juice
- A pinch of black pepper
- 3 tablespoons olive oil
- 2 tablespoons cilantro, chopped

Directions:

1. Arrange the asparagus n a lined baking sheet, add the pesto and the other ingredients, toss, introduce in the oven and cook at 400 degrees F for 20 minutes.
2. Divide between plates and serve as a side dish.

Nutrition facts per serving: calories 114, fat 10.7, fiber 2.4, carbs 4.6, protein 2.6

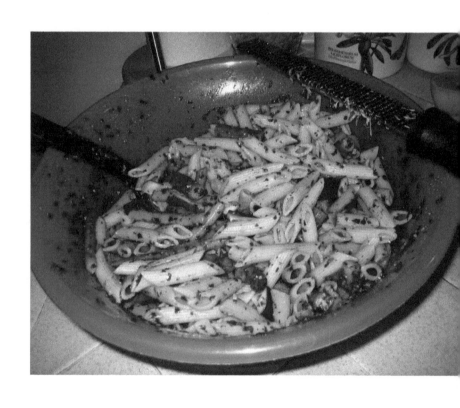

Paprika and Sesame Carrots

Prep time: 10 minutes I **Cooking time:** 30 minutes I

Servings: 4

Ingredients:

- 1 pound baby carrots, trimmed
- 1 tablespoon sweet paprika
- 1 teaspoon lime juice
- 3 tablespoons olive oil
- A pinch of black pepper
- 1 teaspoon sesame seeds

Directions:

1. Arrange the carrots on a lined baking sheet, add the paprika and the other ingredients except the sesame seeds, toss, introduce in the oven and bake at 400 degrees F for 30 minutes.
2. Divide the carrots between plates, sprinkle sesame seeds on top and serve as a side dish.

Nutrition facts per serving: calories 142, fat 11.3, fiber 4.1, carbs 11.4, protein 1.2

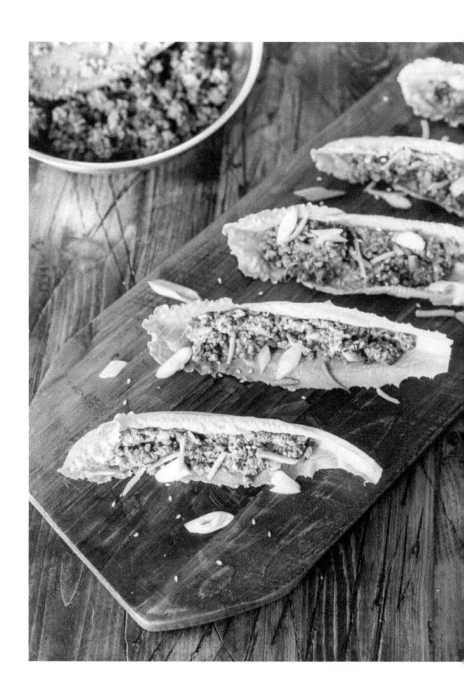

Creamy Parmesan Potato

Prep time: 10 minutes I **Cooking time:** 1 hour I

Servings: 8

Ingredients:

- 1 pound gold potatoes, peeled and cut into wedges
- 2 tablespoons olive oil
- 1 red onion, chopped
- 2 garlic cloves, minced
- 2 cups coconut cream
- 1 tablespoon thyme, chopped
- ¼ teaspoon nutmeg, ground
- ½ cup parmesan, grated

Directions:

1. Heat up a pan with the oil over medium heat, add the onion and the garlic and sauté for 5 minutes.
2. Add the potatoes and brown them for 5 minutes more.
3. Add the cream and the rest of the ingredients, toss gently, bring to a simmer and cook over medium heat for 40 minutes more.
4. Divide the mix between plates and serve as a side dish.

Nutrition facts per serving: calories 230, fat 19.1 fiber 3.3, carbs 14.3, protein 3.6

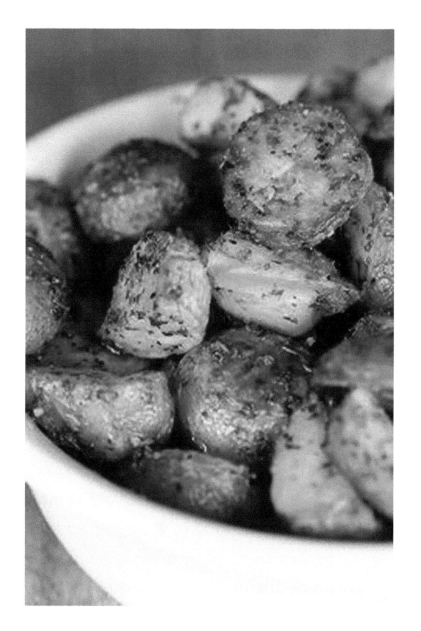

Cabbage Pan

Prep time: 10 minutes I **Cooking time:** 20 minutes I

Servings: 4

Ingredients:

- 1 pound green cabbage, roughly shredded
- 2 tablespoons olive oil
- A pinch of black pepper
- 1 shallot, chopped
- 2 garlic cloves, minced
- 2 tablespoons balsamic vinegar
- 2 teaspoons hot paprika
- 1 teaspoon sesame seeds

Directions:

1. Heat up a pan with the oil over medium heat, add the shallot and the garlic and sauté for 5 minutes.
2. Add the cabbage and the other ingredients, toss, cook over medium heat for 15 minutes, divide between plates and serve.

Nutrition facts per serving: calories 101, fat 7.6, fiber 3.4, carbs 84, protein 1.9

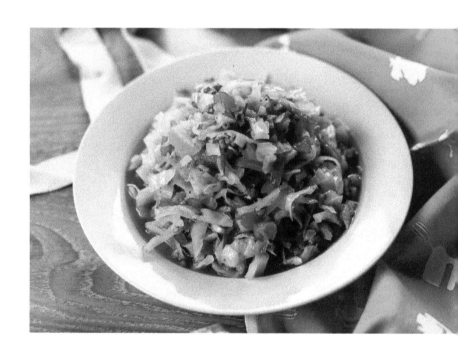

Cilantro and Chili Broccoli

Prep time: 10 minutes I **Cooking time:** 30 minutes I

Servings: 4

Ingredients:

- 2 tablespoons olive oil
- 1 pound broccoli florets
- 2 garlic cloves, minced
- 2 tablespoons chili sauce
- 1 tablespoon lemon juice
- A pinch of black pepper
- 2 tablespoons cilantro, chopped

Directions:

1. In a baking pan, combine the broccoli with the oil, garlic and the other ingredients, toss a bit, introduce in the oven and bake at 400 degrees F for 30 minutes.
2. Divide the mix between plates and serve as a side dish.

Nutrition facts per serving: calories 103, fat 7.4, fiber 3, carbs 8.3, protein 3.4

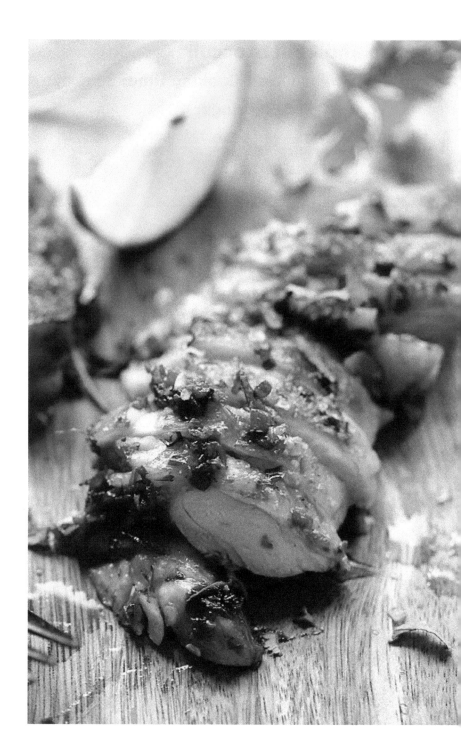

Mozzarella Brussels Sprouts

Prep time: 10 minutes I **Cooking time:** 25 minutes I

Servings: 4

Ingredients:

- 1 tablespoon olive oil
- 1 pound Brussels sprouts, trimmed and halved
- 2 garlic cloves, minced
- ½ cup mozzarella, shredded
- A pinch of pepper flakes, crushed

Directions:

1. In a baking dish, combine the sprouts with the oil and the other ingredients except the cheese and toss.
2. Sprinkle the cheese on top, introduce in the oven and bake at 400 degrees F for 25 minutes.
3. Divide between plates and serve as a side dish.

Nutrition facts per serving: calories 91, fat 4.5, fiber 4.3, carbs 10.9, protein 5

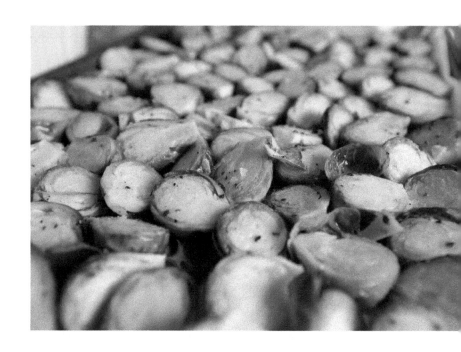

Paprika Brussels Sprouts

Prep time: 10 minutes I **Cooking time:** 25 minutes I

Servings: 4

Ingredients:

- 2 tablespoons olive oil
- 1 pound Brussels sprouts, trimmed and halved
- 3 green onions, chopped
- 2 garlic cloves, minced
- 1 tablespoon balsamic vinegar
- 1 tablespoon sweet paprika
- A pinch of black pepper

Directions:

1. In a baking pan, combine the Brussels sprouts with the oil and the other ingredients, toss and bake at 400 degrees F for 25 minutes.
2. Divide the mix between plates and serve.

Nutrition facts per serving: calories 121, fat 7.6, fiber 5.2, carbs 12.7, protein 4.4

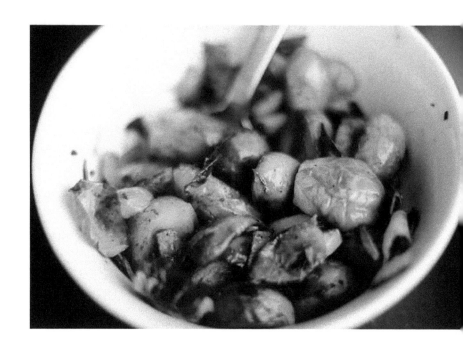

Creamy Cauliflower Mash

Prep time: 10 minutes I **Cooking time:** 25 minutes I

Servings: 4

Ingredients:

- 2 pounds cauliflower florets
- ½ cup coconut milk
- A pinch of black pepper
- ½ cup sour cream
- 1 tablespoon cilantro, chopped
- 1 tablespoon chives, chopped

Directions:

1. Put the cauliflower in a pot, add water to cover, bring to a boil over medium heat, cook for 25 minutes and drain.
2. Mash the cauliflower, add the milk, black pepper and the cream, whisk well, divide between plates, sprinkle the rest of the ingredients on top and serve.

Nutrition facts per serving: calories 188, fat 13.4, fiber 6.4, carbs 15, protein 6.1

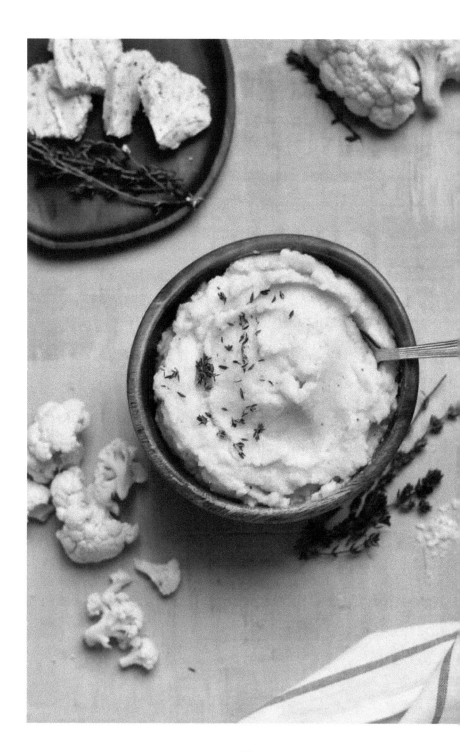

Avocado, Arugula and Olives Salad

Prep time: 5 minutes I **Cooking time:** 0 minutes I

Servings: 4

Ingredients:

- 2 tablespoons olive oil
- 2 avocados, peeled, pitted and cut into wedges
- 1 cup kalamata olives, pitted and halved
- 1 cup tomatoes, cubed
- 1 tablespoon ginger, grated
- A pinch of black pepper
- 2 cups baby arugula
- 1 tablespoon balsamic vinegar

Directions:

1. In a bowl, combine the avocados with the kalamata and the other ingredients, toss and serve as a side dish.

Nutrition facts per serving: calories 320, fat 30.4, fiber 8.7, carbs 13.9, protein 3

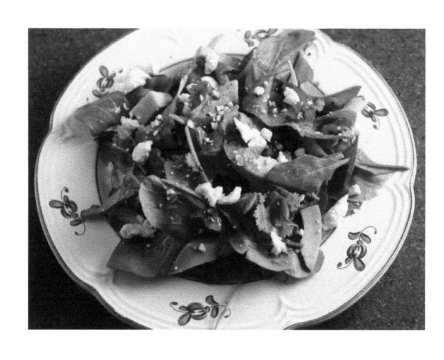

Radish and Olives Salad

Prep time: 5 minutes I **Cooking time:** 0 minutes I

Servings: 4

Ingredients:

- 2 green onions, sliced
- 1 pound radishes, cubed
- 2 tablespoons balsamic vinegar
- 2 tablespoon olive oil
- 1 teaspoon chili powder
- 1 cup black olives, pitted and halved
- A pinch of black pepper

Directions:

1. In a large salad bowl, combine radishes with the onions and the other ingredients, toss and serve as a side dish.

Nutrition facts per serving: calories 123, fat 10.8, fiber 3.3, carbs 7, protein 1.3

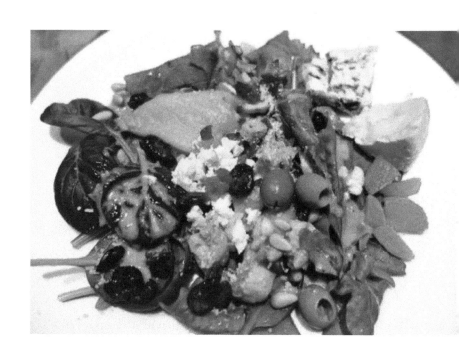

Lemony Endives and Cucumber Salad

Prep time: 5 minutes I **Cooking time:** 0 minutes I

Servings: 4

Ingredients:

- 2 endives, roughly shredded
- 1 tablespoon dill, chopped
- ¼ cup lemon juice
- ¼ cup olive oil
- 2 cups baby spinach
- 2 tomatoes, cubed
- 1 cucumber, sliced
- ½ cups walnuts, chopped

Directions:

1. In a large bowl, combine the endives with the spinach and the other ingredients, toss and serve as a side dish.

Nutrition facts per serving: calories 238, fat 22.3, fiber 3.1, carbs 8.4, protein 5.7

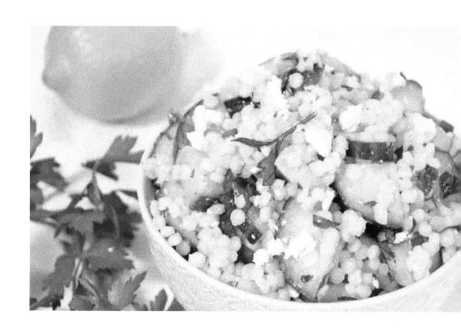

Jalapeno Corn Mix

Prep time: 5 minutes I **Cooking time:** 0 minutes I

Servings: 4

Ingredients:

- 2 tablespoons olive oil
- 1 tablespoon balsamic vinegar
- A pinch of black pepper
- 4 cups corn
- 2 cups black olives, pitted and halved
- 1 red onion, chopped
- ½ cup cherry tomatoes, halved
- 1 tablespoon basil, chopped
- 1 tablespoon jalapeno, chopped
- 2 cups romaine lettuce, shredded

Directions:

1. In a large bowl, combine the corn with the olives, lettuce and the other ingredients, toss well, divide between plates and serve as a side dish.

Nutrition facts per serving: calories 290, fat 16.1, fiber 7.4, carbs 37.6, protein 6.2

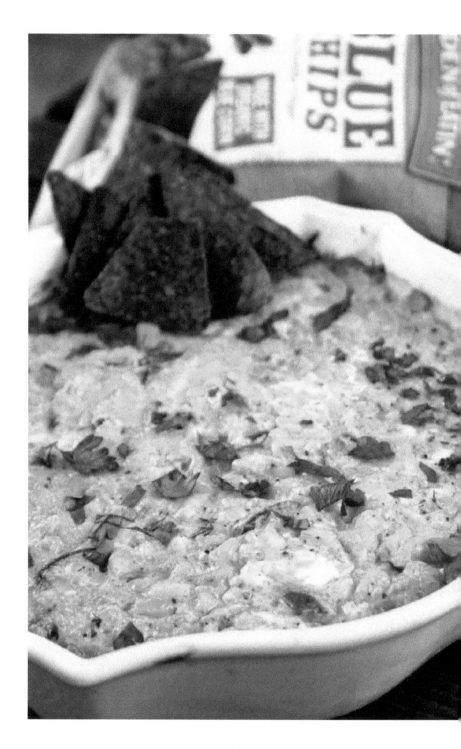

Arugula and Pomegranate Salad

Prep time: 5 minutes I **Cooking time:** 0 minutes I

Servings: 4

Ingredients:

- ¼ cup pomegranate seeds
- 5 cups baby arugula
- 6 tablespoons green onions, chopped
- 1 tablespoon balsamic vinegar
- 2 tablespoons olive oil
- 3 tablespoons pine nuts
- ½ shallot, chopped

Directions:

1. In a salad bowl, combine the arugula with the pomegranate and the other ingredients, toss and serve.

Nutrition facts per serving: calories 120, fat 11.6, fiber 0.9, carbs 4.2, protein 1.8

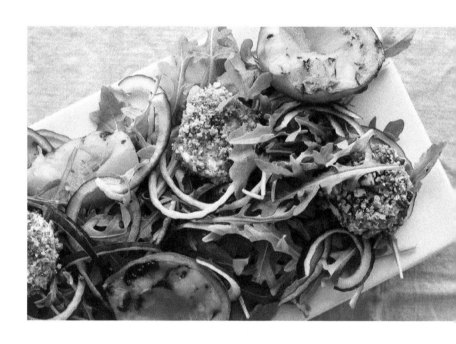

Spinach Mix

Prep time: 10 minutes I **Cooking time:** 0 minutes I

Servings: 4

Ingredients:

- 2 tablespoons olive oil
- 2 avocados, peeled, pitted and cut into wedges
- 3 cups baby spinach
- ¼ cup almonds, toasted and chopped
- 1 tablespoon lemon juice
- 1 tablespoon cilantro, chopped

Directions:

1. In a bowl, combine the avocados with the almonds, spinach and the other ingredients, toss and serve as a side dish.

Nutrition facts per serving: calories 181, fat 4, fiber 4.8, carbs 11.4, protein 6

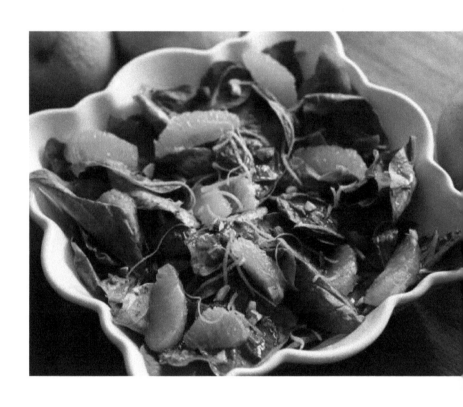

Green Beans and Lettuce Salad

Prep time: 4 minutes I **Cooking time:** 0 minutes I

Servings: 4

Ingredients:

- Juice of 1 lime
- 2 cups romaine lettuce, shredded
- 1 cup corn
- ½ pound green beans, blanched and halved
- 1 cucumber, chopped
- 1/3 cup chives, chopped

Directions:

1. In a bowl, combine the green beans with the corn and the other ingredients, toss and serve.

Nutrition facts per serving: calories 225, fat 12, fiber 2.4, carbs 11.2, protein 3.5

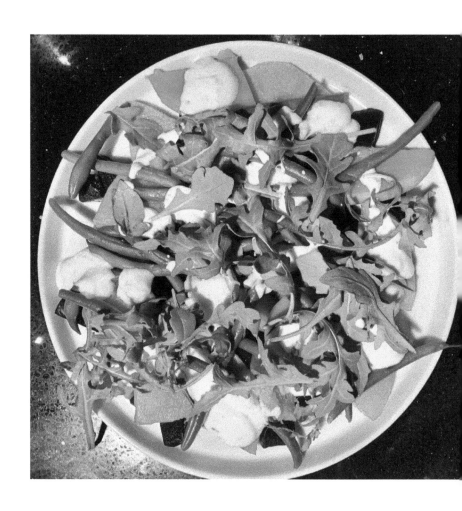

Endives and Onion Salad

Prep time: 4 minutes I **Cooking time:** 0 minutes I

Servings: 4

Ingredients:

- 3 tablespoons olive oil
- 2 endives, trimmed and shredded
- 2 tablespoons lime juice
- 1 tablespoon lime zest, grated
- 1 red onion, sliced
- 1 tablespoon balsamic vinegar
- 1 pound kale, torn
- A pinch of black pepper

Directions:

1. In a bowl, combine the endives with the kale and the other ingredients, toss well and serve cold as a side salad.

Nutrition facts per serving: calories 270, fat 11.4, fiber 5, carbs 14.3, protein 5.7

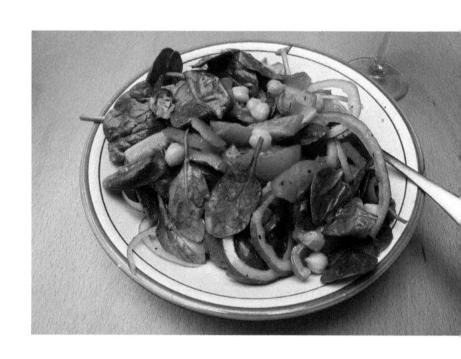

Garlic Edamame

Prep time: 5 minutes I **Cooking time:** 6 minutes I

Servings: 4

Ingredients:

- 2 tablespoons olive oil
- 2 tablespoons balsamic vinegar
- 2 garlic cloves, minced
- 3 cups edamame, shelled
- 1 tablespoon chives, chopped
- 2 shallots, chopped

Directions:

1. Heat up a pan with the oil over medium heat, add the edamame, the garlic and the other ingredients, toss, cook for 6 minutes, divide between plates and serve.

Nutrition facts per serving: calories 270, fat 8.4, fiber 5.3, carbs 11.4, protein 6

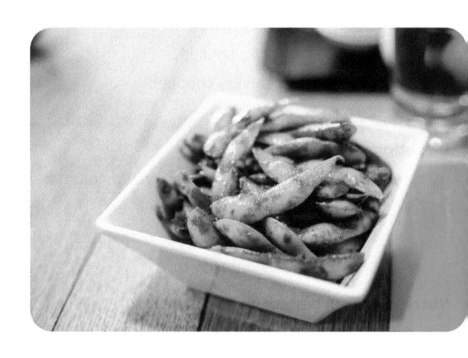

Grapes and Spinach Salad

Prep time: 5 minutes I **Cooking time:** 0 minutes I

Servings: 4

Ingredients:

- 2 cups baby spinach
- 2 avocados, peeled, pitted and roughly cubed
- 1 cucumber, sliced
- 1 and ½ cups green grapes, halved
- 2 tablespoons avocado oil
- 1 tablespoon cider vinegar
- 2 tablespoons parsley, chopped
- A pinch of black pepper

Directions:

1. In a salad bowl, combine the baby spinach with the avocados and the other ingredients, toss and serve.

Nutrition facts per serving: calories 277, fat 11.4, fiber 5, carbs 14.6, protein 4

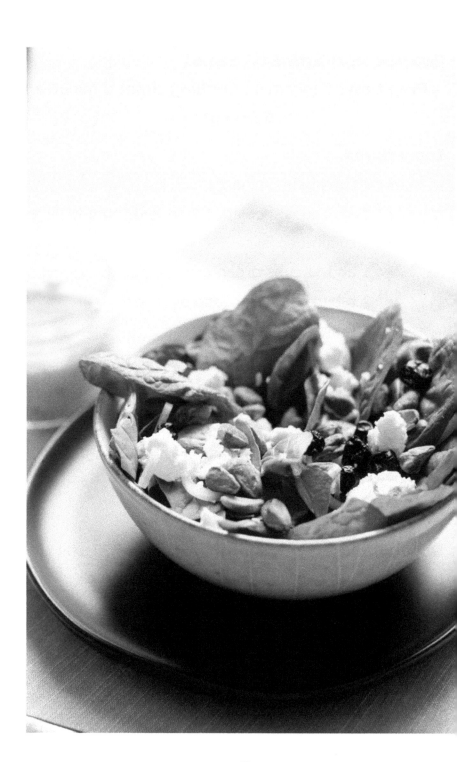

Parmesan Eggplant Mix

Prep time: 10 minutes I **Cooking time:** 20 minutes I

Servings: 4

Ingredients:

- 2 big eggplants, roughly cubed
- 1 tablespoon oregano, chopped
- ½ cup parmesan, grated
- ¼ teaspoon garlic powder
- 2 tablespoons olive oil
- A pinch of black pepper

Directions:

1. In a baking pan combine the eggplants with the oregano and the other ingredients except the cheese and toss.
2. Sprinkle parmesan on top, introduce in the oven and bake at 370 degrees F for 20 minutes.
3. Divide between plates and serve as a side dish.

Nutrition facts per serving: calories 248, fat 8.4, fiber 4, carbs 14.3, protein 5.4

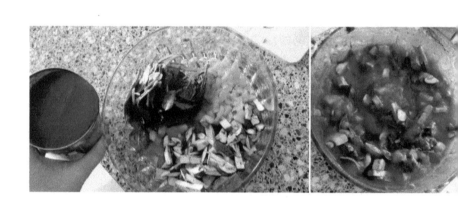

Parmesan Garlic Tomatoes Mix

Prep time: 10 minutes I **Cooking time:** 20 minutes I

Servings: 4

Ingredients:

- 2 pounds tomatoes, halved
- 1 tablespoon basil, chopped
- 3 tablespoons olive oil
- Zest of 1 lemon, grated
- 3 garlic cloves, minced
- ¼ cup parmesan, grated
- A pinch of black pepper

Directions:

1. In a baking pan, combine the tomatoes with the basil and the other ingredients except the cheese and toss.
2. Sprinkle the parmesan on top, introduce in the oven at 375 degrees F for 20 minutes, divide between plates and serve as a side dish.

Nutrition facts per serving: calories 224, fat 12, fiber 4.3, carbs 10.8, protein 5.1

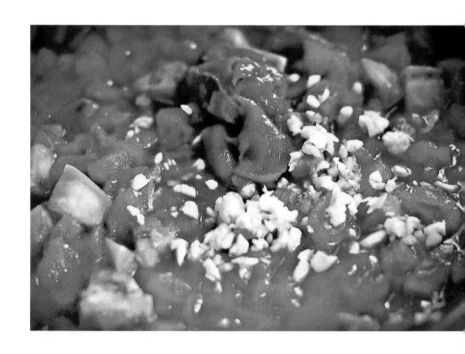

Parsley Mushrooms

Prep time: 10 minutes I **Cooking time:** 30 minutes I

Servings: 4

Ingredients:

- 2 pounds white mushrooms, halved
- 4 garlic cloves, minced
- 2 tablespoons olive oil
- 1 tablespoon thyme, chopped
- 2 tablespoons parsley, chopped
- Black pepper to the taste

Directions:

1. In a baking pan, combine the mushrooms with the garlic and the other ingredients, toss, introduce in the oven and cook at 400 degrees F for 30 minutes.
2. Divide between plates and serve as a side dish.

Nutrition facts per serving: calories 251, fat 9.3, fiber 4, carbs 13.2, protein 6

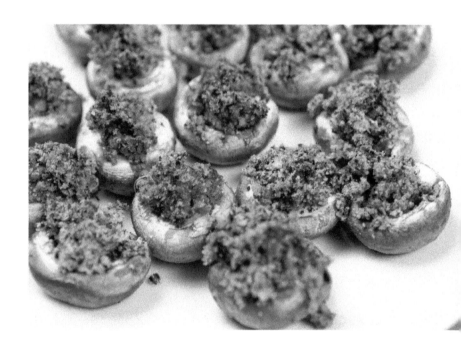

Spinach and Basil Sauté

Prep time: 10 minutes I **Cooking time:** 15 minutes I

Servings: 4

Ingredients:

- 1 cup corn
- 1 pound spinach leaves
- 1 teaspoon sweet paprika
- 1 tablespoon olive oil
- 1 yellow onion, chopped
- ½ cup basil, torn
- A pinch of black pepper
- ½ teaspoon red pepper flakes

Directions:

1. Heat up a pan with the oil over medium-high heat, add the onion, stir and sauté for 5 minutes.
2. Add the corn, spinach and the other ingredients, toss, cook over medium heat for 10 minutes more, divide between plates and serve.

Nutrition facts per serving: calories 201, fat 13.1, fiber 2.5, carbs 14.4, protein 3.7

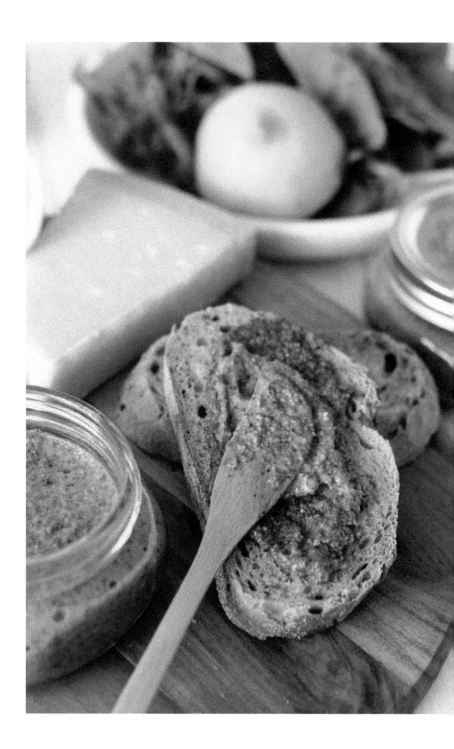

Corn and Shallots Mix

Prep time: 10 minutes I **Cooking time:** 15 minutes I

Servings: 4

Ingredients:

- 4 cups corn
- 1 tablespoon avocado oil
- 2 shallots, chopped
- 1 teaspoon chili powder
- 2 tablespoons tomato pasta
- 3 scallions, chopped
- A pinch of black pepper

Directions:

1. Heat up a pan with the oil over medium-high heat, add the scallions and chili powder, stir and sauté for 5 minutes.
2. Add the corn and the other ingredients, toss, cook for 10 minutes more, divide between plates and serve as a side dish.

Nutrition facts per serving: calories 259, fat 11.1, fiber 2.6, carbs 13.2, protein 3.5

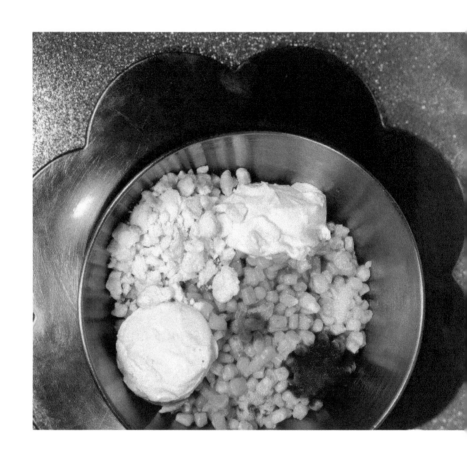

Spinach, Almonds and Capers Salad

Prep time: 10 minutes I **Cooking time:** 0 minutes I

Servings: 4

Ingredients:

- 1 cup mango, peeled and cubed
- 4 cups baby spinach
- 1 tablespoon olive oil
- 2 spring onions, chopped
- 1 tablespoon lemon juice
- 1 tablespoon capers
- 1/3 cup almonds, chopped

Directions:

1. In a bowl, mix the spinach with the mango an d the other ingredients, toss and serve.

Nutrition facts per serving: calories 200, fat 7.4, fiber 3, carbs 4.7, protein 4.4

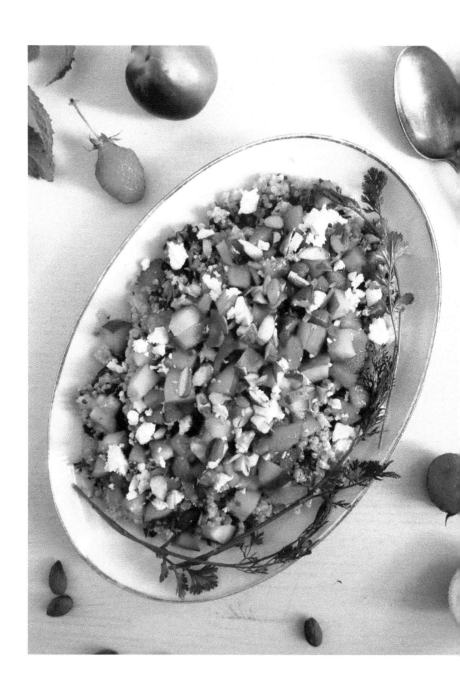

Mustard and Rosemary Potatoes

Prep time: 5 minutes I **Cooking time:** 1 hour I

Servings: 4

Ingredients:

- 1 pound gold potatoes, peeled and cut into wedges
- 2 tablespoons olive oil
- A pinch of black pepper
- 2 tablespoons rosemary, chopped
- 1 tablespoon Dijon mustard
- 2 garlic cloves, minced

Directions:

1. In a baking pan, combine the potatoes with the oil and the other ingredients, toss, introduce in the oven at 400 degrees F and bake for about 1 hour.
2. Divide between plates and serve as a side dish right away.

Nutrition facts per serving: calories 237, fat 11.5, fiber 6.4, carbs 14.2, protein 9

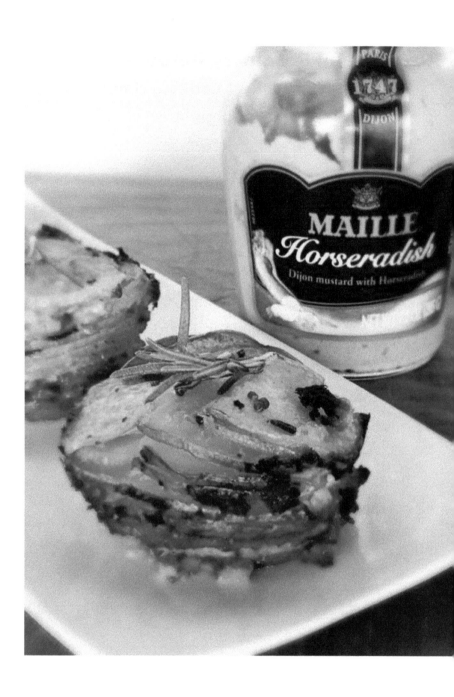

Cashew Brussels Sprouts

Prep time: 5 minutes I **Cooking time:** 30 minutes I

Servings: 4

Ingredients:

- 1 pound Brussels sprouts, trimmed and halved
- 1 cup coconut cream
- 1 tablespoon olive oil
- 2 shallots, chopped
- A pinch of black pepper
- ½ cup cashews, chopped

Directions:

1. In a roasting pan, combine the sprouts with the cream and the rest of the ingredients, toss, and bake in the oven for 30 minutes at 350 degrees F.
2. Divide between plates and serve as a side dish.

Nutrition facts per serving: calories 270, fat 6.5, fiber 5.3, carbs 15.9, protein 3.4

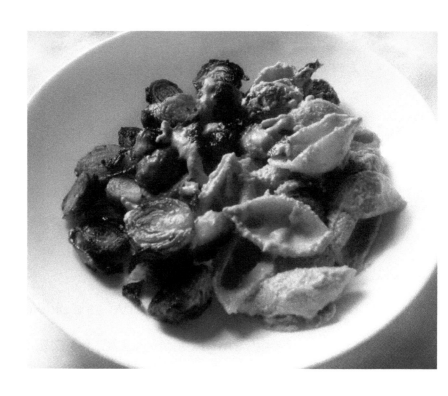

Carrots and Onion Mix

Prep time: 10 minutes I **Cooking time:** 30 minutes I

Servings: 4

Ingredients:

- 2 tablespoons olive oil
- 2 teaspoons sweet paprika
- 1 pound carrots, peeled and roughly cubed
- 1 red onion, chopped
- 1 tablespoon sage, chopped
- A pinch of black pepper

Directions:

1. In a baking pan, combine the carrots with the oil and the other ingredients, toss and bake at 380 degrees F for 30 minutes.
2. Divide between plates and serve.

Nutrition facts per serving: calories 200, fat 8.7, fiber 2.5, carbs 7.9, protein 4

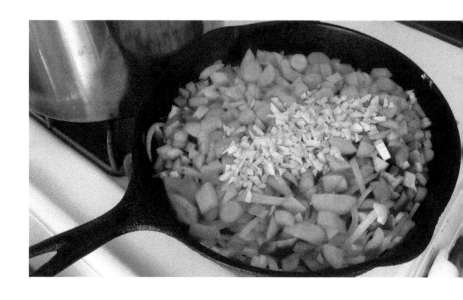

Garlic Mushrooms

Prep time: 10 minutes I **Cooking time:** 20 minutes I

Servings: 4

Ingredients:

- 1 pound white mushrooms, halved
- 2 cups corn
- 2 tablespoons olive oil
- 4 garlic cloves, minced
- 1 cup tomatoes, chopped
- A pinch of black pepper
- ½ teaspoon chili powder

Directions:

1. Heat up a pan with the oil over medium heat, add the mushrooms, garlic and the corn, stir and sauté for 10 minutes.
2. Add the rest of the ingredients, toss, cook over medium heat for 10 minutes more, divide between plates and serve.

Nutrition facts per serving: calories 285, fat 13, fiber 2.2, carbs 14.6, protein 6.7.

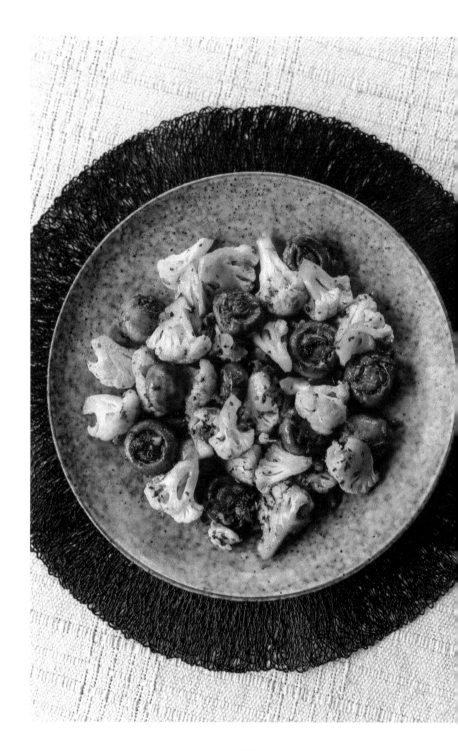

Pesto Green Beans

Prep time: 10 minutes I **Cooking time:** 15 minutes I

Servings: 4

Ingredients:

- 2 tablespoons basil pesto
- 2 teaspoons sweet paprika
- 1 pound green beans, trimmed and halved
- Juice of 1 lemon
- 2 tablespoons olive oil
- 1 red onion, sliced
- A pinch of black pepper

Directions:

1. Heat up a pan with the oil over medium-high heat, add the onion, stir and sauté for 5 minutes.
2. Add the beans and the rest of the ingredients, toss, cook over medium heat for 10 minutes, divide between plates and serve.

Nutrition facts per serving: calories 280, fat 10, fiber 7.6, carbs 13.9, protein 4.7

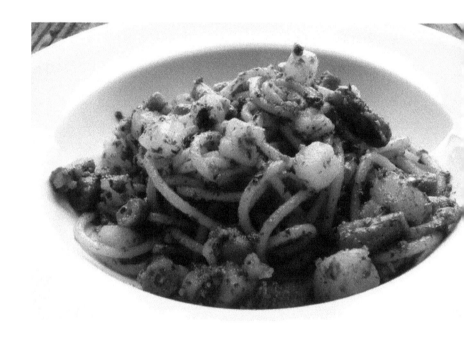

Tarragon and Lime Tomatoes

Prep time: 5 minutes I **Cooking time:** 0 minutes I

Servings: 4

Ingredients:

- 1 and ½ tablespoon olive oil
- 1 pound tomatoes, cut into wedges
- 1 tablespoon lime juice
- 1 tablespoon lime zest, grated
- 2 tablespoons tarragon, chopped
- A pinch of black pepper

Directions:

1. In a bowl, combine the tomatoes with the other ingredients, toss and serve as a side salad.

Nutrition facts per serving: calories 170, fat 4, fiber 2.1, carbs 11.8, proteins 6

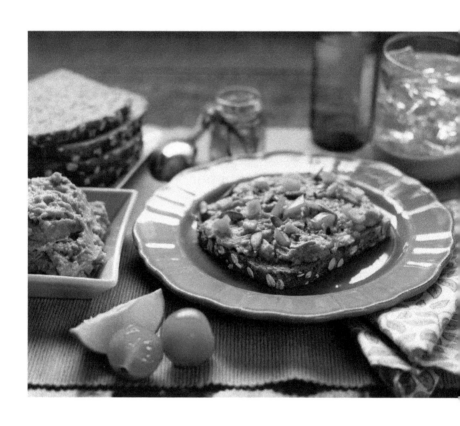

Parsley Beets

Prep time: 10 minutes I **Cooking time:** 30 minutes I

Servings: 4

Ingredients:

- 4 beets, peeled and cut into wedges
- 3 tablespoons olive oil
- 2 tablespoons almonds, chopped
- 2 tablespoons balsamic vinegar
- A pinch of black pepper
- 2 tablespoons parsley, chopped

Directions:

1. In a baking pan, combine the beets with the oil and the other ingredients, toss, introduce in the oven and bake at 400 degrees F for 30 minutes.
2. Divide the mix between plates and serve.

Nutrition facts per serving: calories 230, fat 11, fiber 4.2, carbs 7.3, protein 3.6

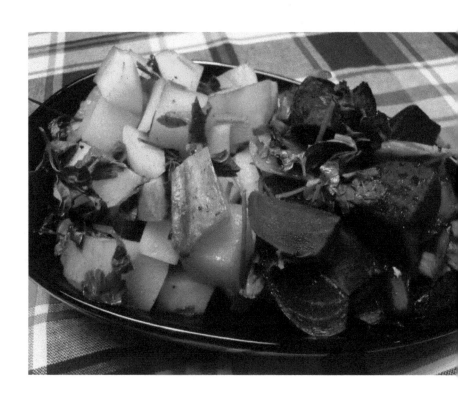

Tomatoes and Vinegar Mix

Prep time: 5 minutes I **Cooking time:** 0 minutes I

Servings: 4

Ingredients:

- 2 tablespoons mint, chopped
- 1 pound tomatoes, cut into wedges
- 2 cups corn
- 2 tablespoons olive oil
- 1 tablespoon rosemary vinegar
- A pinch of black pepper

Directions:

1. In a salad bowl, combine the tomatoes with the corn and the other ingredients, toss and serve.

Nutrition facts per serving: calories 230, fat 7.2, fiber 2, carbs 11.6, protein 4

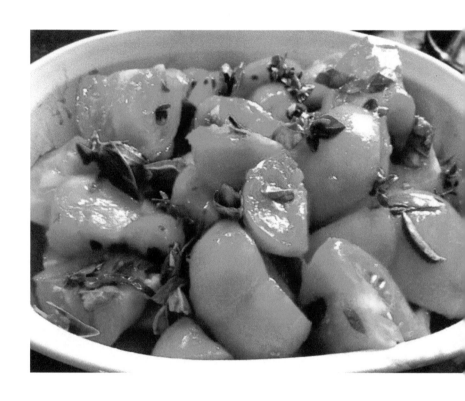

Zucchini Salsa

Prep time: 5 minutes I **Cooking time:** 10 minutes I

Servings: 4

Ingredients:

- 2 tablespoons olive oil
- 2 zucchinis, cubed
- 1 avocado, peeled, pitted and cubed
- 2 tomatoes, cubed
- 1 cucumber, cubed
- 1 yellow onion, chopped
- 2 tablespoons fresh lime juice
- 2 tablespoons cilantro, chopped

Directions:

1. Heat up a pan with the oil over medium heat, add the onion and the zucchinis, toss and cook for 5 minutes.
2. Add the rest of the ingredients, toss, cook for 5 minutes more, divide between plates and serve.

Nutrition facts per serving: calories 290, fat 11.2, fiber 6.1, carbs 14.7, protein 5.6

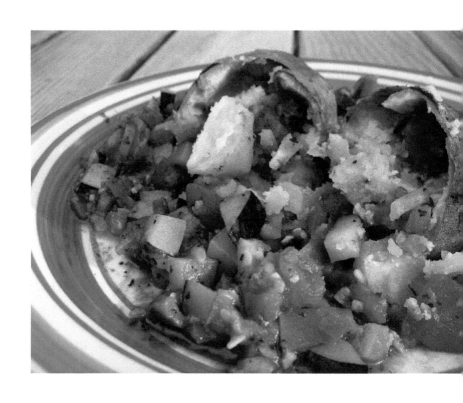

Caraway Cabbage Mix

Prep time: 5 minutes I **Cooking time:** 0 minutes I

Servings: 4

Ingredients:

- 2 green apples, cored and cubed
- 1 red cabbage head, shredded
- 2 tablespoons balsamic vinegar
- ½ teaspoon caraway seeds
- 2 tablespoons olive oil
- Black pepper to the taste

Directions:

1. In a bowl, combine the cabbage with the apples and the other ingredients, toss and serve as a side salad.

Nutrition facts per serving: calories 165, fat 7.4, fiber 7.3, carbs 26, protein 2.6

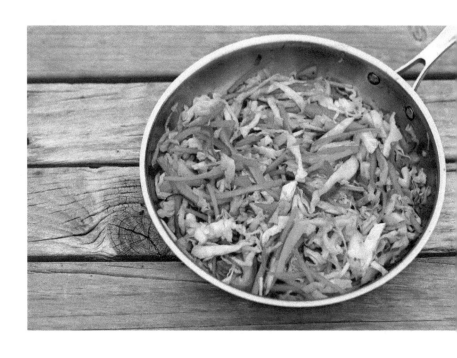

Baked Beets

Prep time: 10 minutes I **Cooking time:** 30 minutes I

Servings: 4

Ingredients:

- 4 beets, peeled and cut into wedges
- 2 tablespoons olive oil
- 2 garlic cloves, minced
- A pinch of black pepper
- ¼ cup parsley, chopped
- ¼ cup walnuts, chopped

Directions:

1. In a baking dish, combine the beets with the oil and the other ingredients, toss to coat, introduce in the oven at 420 degrees F, bake for 30 minutes, divide between plates and serve as a side dish.

Nutrition facts per serving: calories 156, fat 11.8, fiber 2.7, carbs 11.5, protein 3.8

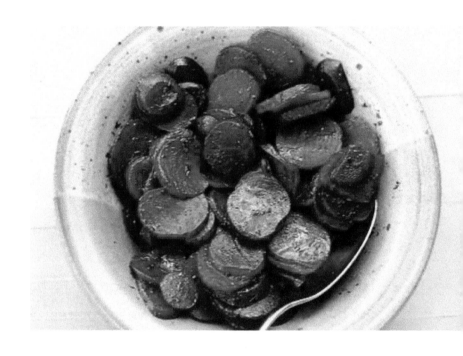

Dill Cabbage and Tomato

Prep time: 10 minutes I **Cooking time:** 15 minutes I

Servings: 4

Ingredients:

- 1 pound green cabbage, shredded
- 1 yellow onion, chopped
- 1 tomato, cubed
- 1 tablespoon dill, chopped
- A pinch of black pepper
- 1 tablespoon olive oil

Directions:

1. Heat up a pan with the oil over medium heat, add the onion and sauté for 5 minutes.
2. Add the cabbage and the rest of the ingredients, toss, cook over medium heat for 10 minutes, divide between plates and serve.

Nutrition facts per serving: calories 74, fat 3.7, fiber 3.7, carbs 10.2, protein 2.1

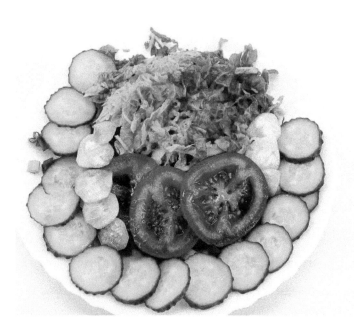

Cabbage and Shallots Salad

Prep time: 5 minutes I **Cooking time:** 0 minutes I

Servings: 4

Ingredients:

- 2 shallots, chopped
- 2 carrots, grated
- 1 big red cabbage head, shredded
- 1 tablespoon olive oil
- 1 tablespoon red vinegar
- A pinch of black pepper
- 1 tablespoon lime juice

Directions:

1. In a bowl, mix the cabbage with the shallots and the other ingredients, toss and serve as a side salad.

Nutrition facts per serving: calories 106, fat 3.8, fiber 6.5, carbs 18, protein 3.3

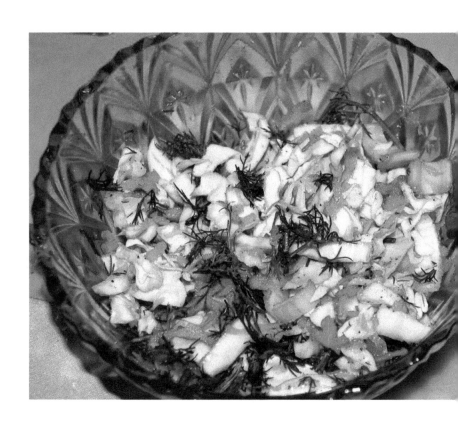

Tomato Salsa

Prep time: 10 minutes I **Cooking time:** 0 minutes I

Servings: 6

Ingredients:

- 1 pound cherry tomatoes, halved
- 2 tablespoons olive oil
- 1 cup kalamata olives, pitted and halved
- A pinch of black pepper
- 1 red onion, chopped
- 1 tablespoon balsamic vinegar
- ¼ cup cilantro, chopped

Directions:

1. In a bowl, mix the tomatoes with the olives and the other ingredients, toss and serve as a side salad.

Nutrition facts per serving: calories 131, fat 10.9, fiber 3.1, carbs 9.2, protein 1.6

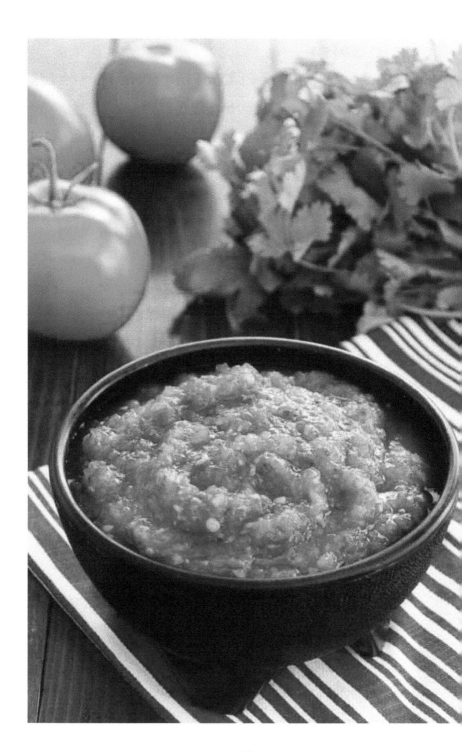

Pesto Zucchini Salad

Prep time: 4 minutes I **Cooking time:** 0 minutes I

Servings: 4

Ingredients:

- 2 zucchinis, cut with a spiralizer
- 1 red onion, sliced
- 1 tablespoon basil pesto
- 1 tablespoon lemon juice
- 1 tablespoon olive oil
- ½ cup cilantro, chopped
- Black pepper to the taste

Directions:

1. In a salad bowl, mix the zucchinis with the onion and the other ingredients, toss and serve.

Nutrition facts per serving: calories 58, fat 3.8, fiber 1.8, carbs 6, protein 1.6

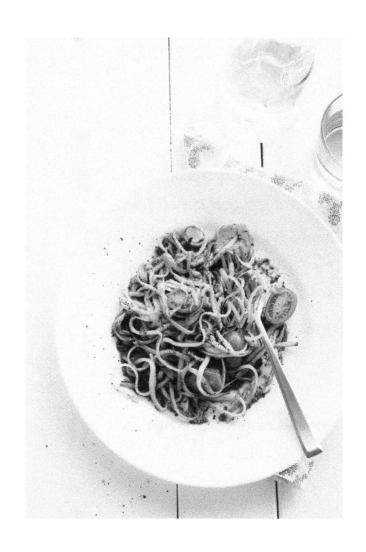

Carrots Slaw

Prep time: 4 minutes I **Cooking time:** 0 minutes I

Servings: 4

Ingredients:

- 1 pound carrots, peeled and roughly grated
- 2 tablespoons avocado oil
- 2 tablespoons lemon juice
- 3 tablespoons sesame seeds
- ½ teaspoon curry powder
- 1 teaspoon rosemary, dried
- ½ teaspoon cumin, ground

Directions:

1. In a bowl, mix the carrots with the oil, lemon juice and the other ingredients, toss and serve cold as a side salad.

Nutrition facts per serving: calories 99, fat 4.4, fiber 4.2, carbs 13.7, protein 2.4

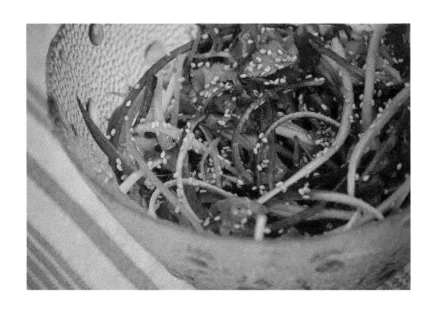

Lettuce Salad

Prep time: 5 minutes I **Cooking time:** 0 minutes I

Servings: 4

Ingredients:

- 1 tablespoon ginger, grated
- 2 garlic cloves, minced
- 4 cups romaine lettuce, torn
- 1 beet, peeled and grated
- 2 green onions, chopped
- 1 tablespoon balsamic vinegar
- 1 tablespoon sesame seeds

Directions:

1. In a bowl, combine the lettuce with the ginger, garlic and the other ingredients, toss and serve as a side dish.

Nutrition facts per serving: calories 42, fat 1.4, fiber 1.5, carbs 6.7, protein 1.4

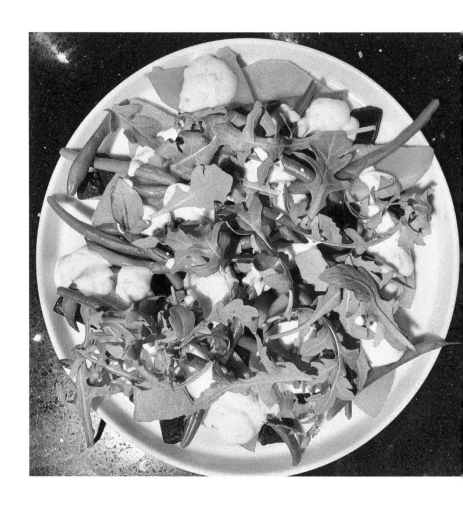

Chives Radishes

Prep time: 5 minutes I **Cooking time:** 0 minutes I

Servings: 4

Ingredients:

- 1 pound red radishes, roughly cubed
- 1 tablespoon chives, chopped
- 1 tablespoon parsley, chopped
- 1 tablespoon oregano, chopped
- 2 tablespoons olive oil
- 1 tablespoon lime juice
- Black pepper to the taste

Directions:

1. In a salad bowl, mix the radishes with the chives and the other ingredients, toss and serve.

Nutrition facts per serving: calories 85, fat 7.3, fiber 2.4, carbs 5.6, protein 1

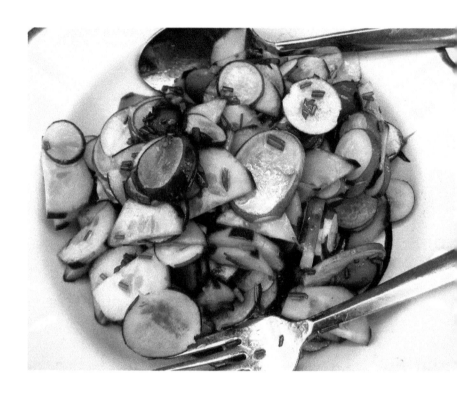

Lime Fennel Mix

Prep time: 5 minutes I **Cooking time:** 20 minutes I

Servings: 4

Ingredients:

- 2 fennel bulbs, sliced
- 1 teaspoon sweet paprika
- 1 small red onion, sliced
- 2 tablespoons olive oil
- 2 tablespoons lime juice
- 2 tablespoons dill, chopped
- Black pepper to the taste

Directions:

1. In a roasting pan, combine the fennel with the paprika and the other ingredients, toss, and bake at 380 degrees F for 20 minutes.
2. Divide the mix between plates and serve.

Nutrition facts per serving: calories 114, fat 7.4, fiber 4.5, carbs 13.2, protein 2.1

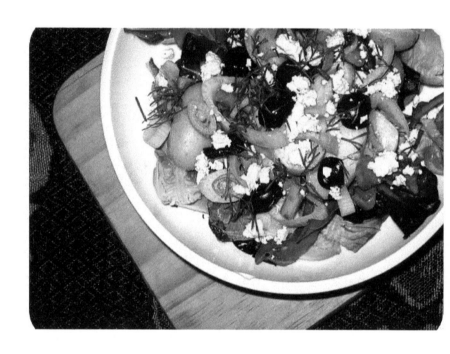

Oregano Peppers

Prep time: 10 minutes I **Cooking time:** 30 minutes I

Servings: 4

Ingredients:

- 1 pound mixed bell peppers, cut into wedges
- 1 red onion, thinly sliced
- 2 tablespoons olive oil
- Black pepper to the taste
- 1 tablespoon oregano, chopped
- 2 tablespoons mint leaves, chopped

Directions:

1. In a roasting pan, combine the bell peppers with the onion and the other ingredients, toss and bake at 380 degrees F for 30 minutes.
2. Divide the mix between plates and serve.

Nutrition facts per serving: calories 240, fat 8.2, fiber 4.2, carbs 11.3, protein 5.6

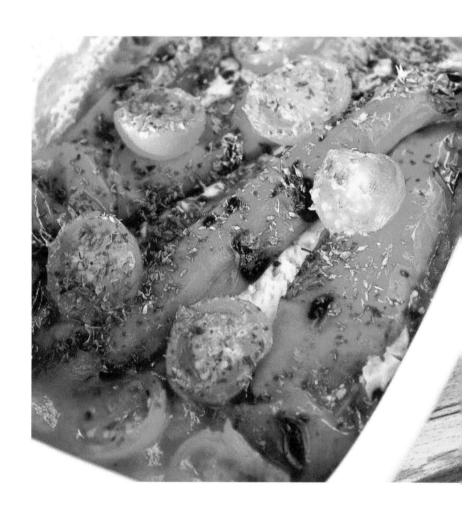

Red Cabbage Sauté

Prep time: 5 minutes I **Cooking time:** 15 minutes I

Servings: 4

Ingredients:

- 1 pound red cabbage, shredded
- 8 dates, pitted and sliced
- 2 tablespoons olive oil
- ¼ cup veggie stock
- 2 tablespoons chives, chopped
- 2 tablespoons lemon juice
- Black pepper to the taste

Directions:

1. Heat up a pan with the oil over medium heat, add the cabbage and the dates, toss and cook for 4 minutes.
2. Add the stock and the other ingredients, toss, cook over medium heat for 11 minutes more, divide between plates and serve.

Nutrition facts per serving: calories 280, fat 8.1, fiber 4.1, carbs 8.7, protein 6.3

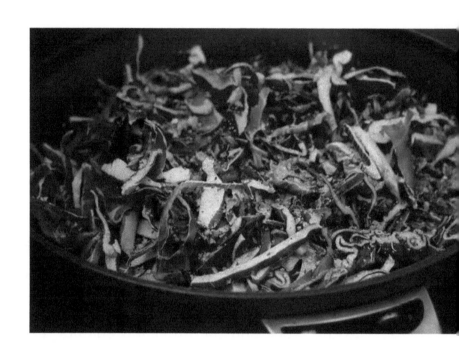

Black Beans and Shallots Mix

Prep time: 4 minutes I **Cooking time:** 0 minutes I

Servings: 4

Ingredients:

- 3 cups black beans, cooked
- 1 cup cherry tomatoes, halved
- 2 shallots, chopped
- 3 tablespoons olive oil
- 1 tablespoon balsamic vinegar
- Black pepper to the taste
- 1 tablespoon chives, chopped

Directions:

1. In a bowl, combine the beans with the tomatoes and the other ingredients, toss and serve cold as a side dish.

Nutrition facts per serving: calories 310, fat 11.0, fiber 5.3, carbs 19.6, protein 6.8

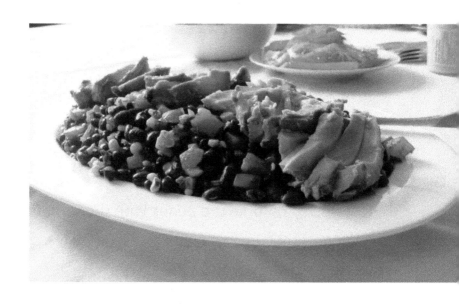

Cilantro Olives Mix

Prep time: 4 minutes I **Cooking time:** 0 minutes I

Servings: 4

Ingredients:

- 2 spring onions, chopped
- 2 endives, shredded
- 1 cup black olives, pitted and sliced
- ½ cup kalamata olives, pitted and sliced
- ¼ cup apple cider vinegar
- 2 tablespoons olive oil
- 1 tablespoons cilantro, chopped

Directions:

1. In a bowl, mix the endives with the olives and the other ingredients, toss and serve.

Nutrition facts per serving: calories 230, fat 9.1, fiber 6.3, carbs 14.6, protein 7.2

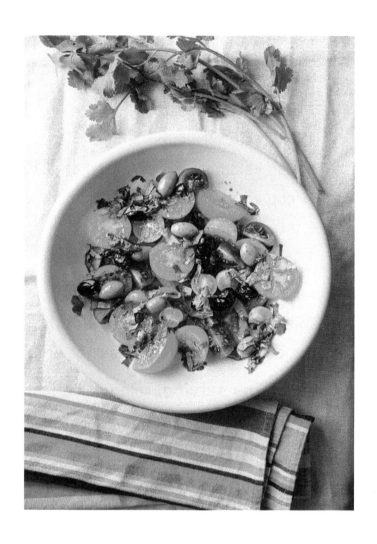

Basil Tomatoes and Cucumber Mix

Prep time: 5 minutes I **Cooking time:** 0 minutes I

Servings: 4

Ingredients:

- ½ pound tomatoes, cubed
- 2 cucumber, sliced
- 1 tablespoon olive oil
- 2 spring onions, chopped
- Black pepper to the taste
- Juice of 1 lime
- ½ cup basil, chopped

Directions:

1. In a salad bowl, combine the tomatoes with the cucumber and the other ingredients, toss and serve cold.

Nutrition facts per serving: calories 224, fat 11.2, fiber 5.1, carbs 8.9, protein 6.2

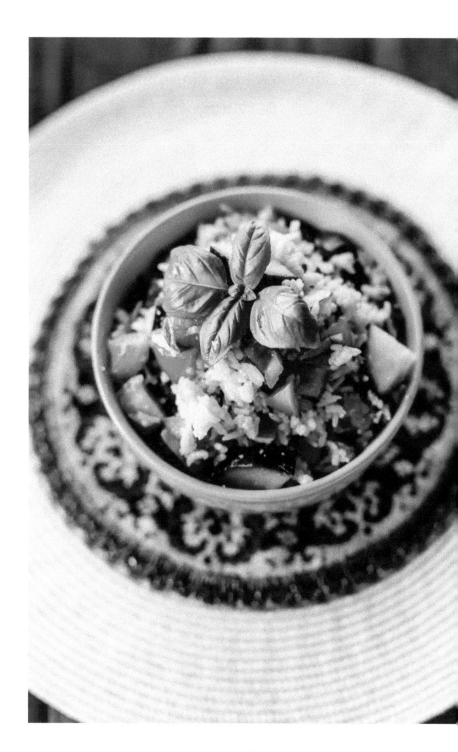

Peppers Salad

Prep time: 5 minutes I **Cooking time:** 0 minutes I

Servings: 4

Ingredients:

- 1 cup cherry tomatoes, halved
- 1 yellow bell pepper, chopped
- 1 red bell pepper, chopped
- 1 green bell pepper, chopped
- ½ pound carrots, shredded
- 3 tablespoons red wine vinegar
- 2 tablespoons olive oil
- 1 tablespoon cilantro, chopped
- Black pepper to the taste

Directions:

1. In a salad bowl, mix the tomatoes with the peppers, carrots and the other ingredients, toss and serve as a side salad.

Nutrition facts per serving: calories 123, fat 4, fiber 8.4, carbs 14.4, protein 1.1

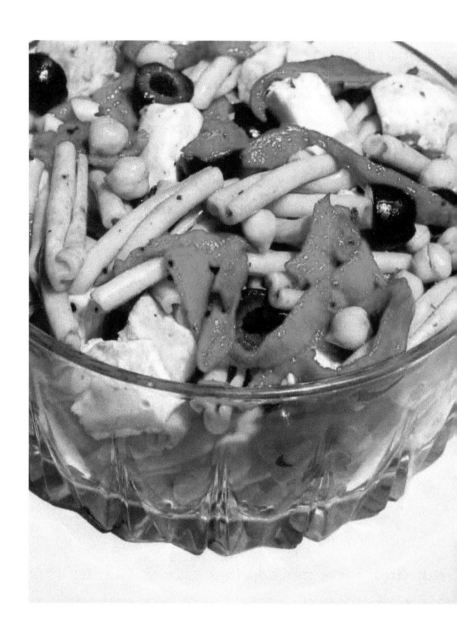

Thyme Rice Mix

Prep time: 10 minutes I **Cooking time:** 30 minutes I
Servings: 4

Ingredients:

- 2 tablespoons olive oil
- 1 yellow onion, chopped
- 1 cup black beans, cooked
- 2 cup black rice
- 4 cups chicken stock
- 2 tablespoons thyme, chopped
- Zest of ½ lemon, grated
- A pinch of black pepper

Directions:

1. Heat up a pan with the oil over medium-high heat, add the onion, stir and sauté for 4 minutes.
2. Add the beans, rice and the other ingredients, toss, bring to a boil and cook over medium heat for 25 minutes.
3. Stir the mix, divide between plates and serve.

Nutrition facts per serving: calories 290, fat 15.3, fiber 6.2, carbs 14.6, protein 8

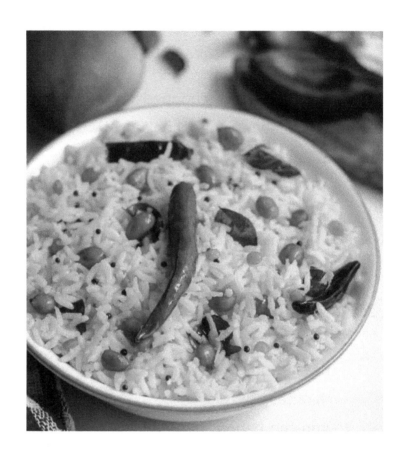

Rice and Cranberries Mix

Prep time: 10 minutes I **Cooking time:** 25 minutes I

Servings: 4

Ingredients:

- 1 cup cauliflower florets
- 1 cup brown rice
- 2 cups chicken stock
- 1 tablespoon avocado oil
- 2 shallots, chopped
- ¼ cup cranberries
- ½ cup almonds, sliced

Directions:

1. Heat up a pan with the oil over medium heat, add the shallots, stir and sauté for 5 minutes.
2. Add the cauliflower, the rice and the other ingredients, toss, bring to a simmer and cook over medium heat for 20 minutes.
3. Divide the mix between plates and serve.

Nutrition facts per serving: calories 290, fat 15.1, fiber 5.6, carbs 7, protein 4.5

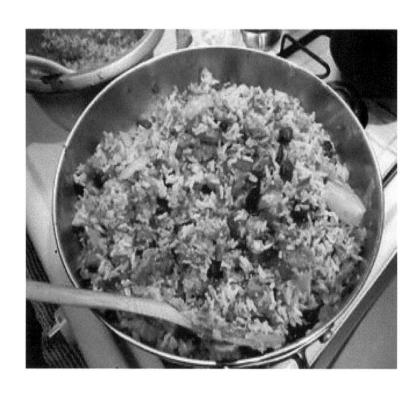

Oregano Beans Salad

Prep time: 10 minutes I **Cooking time:** 0 minutes I

Servings: 4

Ingredients:

- 2 cups black beans, cooked
- 2 cups white beans, cooked
- 2 tablespoons balsamic vinegar
- 2 tablespoons olive oil
- 1 teaspoon oregano, dried
- 1 teaspoon basil, dried
- 1 tablespoon chives, chopped

Directions:

1. In a salad bowl, combine the beans with the vinegar and the other ingredients, toss and serve as a side salad.

Nutrition facts per serving: calories 322, fat 15.1, fiber 10, carbs 22.0, protein 7

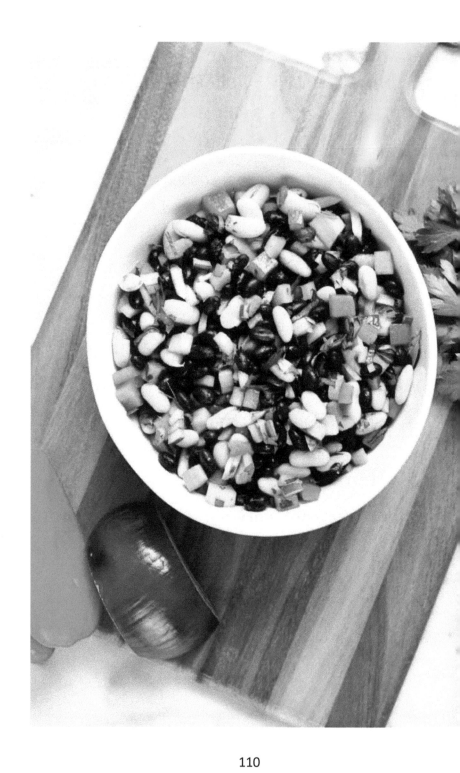

Lightning Source UK Ltd.
Milton Keynes UK
UKHW020626140621
385475UK00001B/138